The Journey

Brad L Horton

ISBN: 1984080741
ISBN-13: 978-1984080745

DEDICATION

This book is dedicated to my wife, Rhonda, who faithfully cared for me; my children, Madison, Cari, Amelia, and Matthew, whose lives were rearranged; and my parents, Ralph and Darresa, who put their lives on hold to help during my treatment. Without these people, I cannot imagine what it would have been like.

CONTENTS

PREFACE

"You have POEMS," the doctor said. "It is a cousin of Multiple Myeloma." I remember the office visit that day and feelings of relief and fear at the same time. Beginning in 2013 through the spring of 2016, I went from diagnosis to deliverance. I am amazed at what God has done through modern medicine. I am amazed that God has chosen to give me more time on this earth.

My sister-in-law, who is an expert writer and editor, encouraged me to write about my experience, so that is exactly what I'm doing. It has taken a while to put things together because of other commitments, jobs, responsibilities, and the day-to-day life events we deal with.

My purpose in writing this book is to share my experience before, during, and after diagnosis. It was a great help to me to find support groups during my treatment, to see what others experienced, to see their path and treatment. I hope this will help someone to press on.

There are many who find themselves with a mountain of issues ahead of them. I faced those mountains as well. Seeing what others endured helped me to face the challenges before me. And not just the physical challenges, but the financial, emotional, and logistical ones as well.

Finally, I just want to share how faith helps. Some

may not believe in God. Some may have doubts. I want to share how my faith in God helped me to manage through some trials. In the end, no amount of modern medicine is possible without God endowing man with the ability to provide it. God has the final say about whether we live or die.

I hope that you will read to be encouraged in your battle. May God grant healing to you if you're in the battle, and may God grant wisdom and peace if you're helping in the battle. Press on.

Something's Not Right

It is always easier to treat the symptom than the problem. We often find ourselves doing that today because it is easier. Go to the doctor, tell him or her the symptom, call in a pill, and you're done. Then when the symptom returns, go back and do the same process again. This is not an attack on the medical professionals we all respect. The truth is many doctors just do this because they don't have the resources or the initiative to dig to find the problem. Where there is smoke, there's fire, always.

My mother-in-law, who died in October of 2013, had symptoms of cancer for a while. It took some time to get to the root of the problem, the issue causing her symptoms. It was during the summer of 2013, the summer she was enduring her battle, that I decided to go to the doctor for a checkup. My mother-in-law was a trouper, a woman who never stopped. She was always on the go, shopping, going to yard sales, selling and buying furniture, or rearranging and replacing furniture in the

1

house. She had never been to the doctor. In fact, the last doctor visit she had was after my wife was born 41 years earlier. Seeing the sickness that had developed in her, I decided I should be looked over. Little did I know the journey this would begin.

In June 2013, I made the appointment to be looked over. Proverbs 27:1 says, *"Do not boast about tomorrow, for you do not know what a day may bring."* This world is unstable. Life itself is unstable. We may predict, suppose, or hope for a day to bring something, but in reality, none of us knows what it brings. No one wants the stock market to go down, but it does. News can bring down a stock quickly, and a man can "lose his shirt" in a moment's notice. For me, what I have learned over this journey is that life can change in a moment. I hope that the process I am about to outline will help you if you are struggling with a disease that no one can figure out. Maybe, by the grace of God, you can find help. I am discovering that many people have died from symptoms similar to POEMS that no one has been able to pinpoint. So here we go. Let me say this, God used my mother-in-law's sickness to get me to the doctor. We all prayed for her to get well, but in the end, her death may have saved my life. Miss you, Nancy Webster.

The Blood Test

My checkup was with an internal doctor near Atlanta, a part of the Emory Health System. Most of us have been through a checkup sometime in our life. Standard examinations, questions, and blood work are normal. All went well, I went to the lab on site, they drew blood, and I went home. I knew from blood tests years ago that I might have had out-of-range bad cholesterol. I expected that to show up.

It was two days later when I received a message on my phone. The message was, "There's an abnormality in your lab work. Please call." Who wants a phone call like that? I called, and no information was given over the phone. I made an appointment for two days later, and that seemed like the longest two days I have ever had. Do you know what goes through a man's mind? Cancer?

After arriving at the doctor's office, I awaited the news of the results. They weren't mind blowing, as I had worked myself up to assume they would be. In fact, it was nothing terribly abnormal. My glucose was a little high, but she noted that I had high hemoglobin and hematocrit. Some of the causes of high hemoglobin are, according to the Mayo Clinic, that, "You smoke or you live at higher altitudes and your red blood cell production naturally increases to compensate for the lower oxygen supply there."

The hematologist I was seeing was a very good and caring and knowledgeable doctor. He has been a doctor a long time and looked puzzled and had no quick answer of why I had this. He began to explain how the kidney works to get blood to the system, and he wanted an ultrasound of my kidney. "Interesting," I thought. So the kidney ultrasound was scheduled for the next week.

The following week, I went to the hematologist and had

basic CBC labs done, still showing high hemoglobin and hematocrit. The doctor came in with results from the kidney ultrasound, and all was normal. There was one interesting comment he made, and looking back now, if he had been familiar with POEMS syndrome, he might have made a note of it, but he didn't. He noted on the report an enlarged spleen, but he wasn't concerned about it. Well, neither was I.

He then spoke the words that sent chills up my spine: "Bone marrow aspiration." I knew that meant getting marrow, and the only place for marrow was in the bone. Yikes! I panicked, called my wife, and was on the verge of tears. It was to be done then, in the office. All right, I said, knowing that maybe this would yield some answers. As I researched the "possibilities" of high hemoglobin and hematocrit, I saw the words "bone marrow dysfunction," and I saw now this may have been the early symptoms of POEMS. That's just my opinion. I waited to be called to the room for the extraction. It was uncomfortable, but I made it. Many others do it far more often than I do, and I know their pain, God bless them.

Two weeks later, I was back at the office for the report and more labs. Those labs showed the same results as before, and the pathology report was what had me on pins and needles. The doctor came in, and the first words out of his mouth were, "Bone marrow is normal" with the exception of this noted in the report: "Slightly hyper-cellular bone marrow with trilineage hematopoiesis." What does that mean? In a nutshell, it was normal. Of course, this was great news. However, we were back to the drawing board. The solution was to have a pint of blood drawn off to reduce the high counts. I assumed that this would be the normal life for me, having some blood drawn off every few months.

Something Not Right In My Toes

I followed up with the internal doctor who did my initial checkup in July of 2013. It was not until November of 2013 when I returned to the doctor for more blood work. The internal medicine doctor knew of the hematologist visit and had all the notes. I mentioned to her that I had some tingling in my feet, some "off" sensations. No pain, no initial discomfort, but something wasn't right. I had noticed during December some knots and pain in the bottom of my left foot. For some reason, I had been developing some weakness. I assumed I was tired. She took a look at my B-12 levels, which were on the low end of normal. I was prescribed B-12 shots. I started those in November of 2013, and by the end of December 2013 I was back at her office. My complaint? Something was still not right. The shots didn't help one bit. I was now unusually tired from the extra effort to walk. The walking had become difficult to a degree.

So far, the little blood test that revealed high hemoglobin and hematocrit had produced nothing, except I was noticing some worsening issues. I had by then decided to see a neurologist. In January of 2014, I made an appointment with a well-known nerve doctor in Atlanta. My appointment was

5

scheduled for the first week of February. It was the first week of January, my feet were developing some shocking, shooting-fire pain, not constant, but my walk had become noticeably awkward.

Now is a good time to mention that my profession is UPS service provider. I am on my feet all day, up and down. In hindsight, this job—the active working daily—helped me go as long as I did before I was literally unable to work.

The day for the neurologist visit came. I was expecting answers. I didn't get them. The doctor was intrigued as well about my diagnosis so far, which was "thick blood." He had the notes and labs from the hematologist as well. He went through a detailed neurologic exam then ordered blood tests. More blood tests? I thought, "What can he know from blood tests? After all, I have been thoroughly examined by a hematologist. He also ordered an EMG, which is a nerve test, sending electric shocks through legs and arms to determine nerve speed. I went to the lab then went home.

The follow-up appointment was also the day of the EMG test. That test lasted nearly two hours, and I felt tortured afterward from all the electrical current. I would not have to wait for the results of this test, as the doctor reads them immediately. After a few minutes of waiting, I heard the doctor arrive and say, "We need some more blood work" and "The EMG is abnormal." Is abnormal bad in this case? Can it be fixed? I didn't get these answers. He said only that we needed to look at other causes. I look back on this conversation and I see the wheels in his brain turning, trying to figure out why I was having these symptoms. Something wasn't normal compared to what he had seen in his profession. He was looking deeper, but I didn't know it.

The Plot Thickens, Literally

There are conversations a man will never forget, and this was one of them. I was working, having just made a delivery, and while on my way back to the truck, the phone rang. It was the neurologist. The conversation went something like this: "All is normal in the blood work, except there's an abnormal protein in your blood called IGG." My response? "Okay." He then says, "I'm going to call your hematologist for some help." To be honest, this didn't sound good. A hematologist has already tried all he knows, and now one of the highest regarded specialists in nerves is calling the hematologist for help.

At the time, he was careful to say what he was suspecting without further investigation, but the fact of the matter was that it was either blood cancer or a blood disorder producing this abnormal protein. As we hung up the phone, I didn't really know what to do. I was perplexed. I finished the remainder of the day somewhat distressed, with no answer yet after months of seeing doctors. On the way home, I received a call from the hematologist around 6:00 p.m., late for a doctor's office, wanting an appointment with me on Monday. This was Thursday. This really sent me over the edge. Why so soon? Did he know something? It was a long weekend.

Sitting in the doctor's office in March of 2014 and waiting for the hematologist to come in was nerve-racking. The doctor came in and addressed the concerns that my neurologist had. He explained in great detail the blood tests such as IGG, IGA, IGM, and B-2 Microglobulin tests. It was fascinating, to say the least, what the blood reveals. He agreed this could—in a very, very unlikely outcome—be Multiple Myeloma. The "very unlikely" message was a bit comforting, but it didn't soothe my nerves. He explained he was going to do more specific blood tests, and some were some kind of genetic blood work as well. An appointment was made for two weeks later, and so I waited, again.

It was now the latter part of March. Back again to the hematologist. As we sat in the waiting room, my wife and I, I was nervous, and she was too, but she never showed it. The doctor came in, and the first words out of his mouth were, "No Myeloma." Glory. He said there was no indication whatsoever of the blood cancer. All other genetic blood tests showed no abnormalities, either, and my hemoglobin and hematocrit were still high. So the treatment was, let's drain some more blood. Really? What now? My feet were going numb, my muscles were getting weak, and drop foot was setting in. We left the office with no more solutions than we began with in July of 2013. It was now March 2014, and we had no solution.

CIDP?

I called the neurologist to schedule a follow-up again with the results from the hematologist. It would be five weeks before I could see him again. That was not acceptable. I prayed for a good neurologist to help. The Lord opened the door for me to see a local neurologist, Dr. David Williams. Most neurologists I have ever seen have been very formal and serious. When Dr. Williams came in, he was wearing an earring and biker boots. My first thought was, really? He was very straight and to the point. He read all the other tests, scans, and blood work results from the former neurologist. After looking at all the data, he came up with what I might have. He called it CIDP, Chronic Inflammatory Demyelinating Polyneuropathy. The diagnosis made sense at the moment. He further added that he needed to confirm this by doing a spinal tap. Yikes! Just the sound of such a procedure sent chills up my spine, no pun intended.

The reason for the tap was to determine if there was an abnormal amount of protein in the spinal fluid. If this was present, it would confirm the diagnosis. Elevated protein levels are common (80% of CIDP patients); 10% of patients also have mild lymphocytic pleocytosis and increased gamma globulin. Enough of the detailed medical terminology.

The procedure was set up for the next week. It was a breeze compared to the bone marrow aspiration. Dr. Williams was brilliant at the procedure. The hardest part of the spinal tap was waiting on the fluid to come out. It takes a while and comes out one drip at a time. It was clear, and that was always good. The wait now began to see what the results showed. At this time, I was hoping for a positive protein so we could get a diagnosis.

9

Less than a week later, Dr. Williams called. "You have very elevated protein in your spinal fluid."

"Okay," I responded.

"You definitely have CIDP," Dr. Williams said. Hearing this was good news because there were treatable options. The first one, which is what I started on in April of 2014, was prednisone, a steroid. I was warned of its side effects—insomnia, weight gain, and some increased energy. I started on 60 milligrams a day.

Initial Results

I was to see Dr. Williams at the end of May 2014 for a follow-up from initial doses of prednisone. At that approximately five-week visit, there was no notable difference, with the exception that I wasn't any worse. On several occasions, I started noticing some swelling in the feet and ankles. Given the fact of nerve issues, I assumed that was the cause. I didn't think much of it. The swelling was never constant. It came and went. The June follow-up showed the same, no changes, nothing better, nothing worse. I was having considerable drop-foot issues now. Off I went to see a foot doctor, and an orthotic was made for my right foot.

The July visit to Dr. Williams once again proved the same. No real changes, no worsening, either. Another EMG was ordered for early August. Arriving at the hospital for the test, and knowing what was coming with all the electrical shocks, I was a bit nervous again. Not even all the way through the procedure, Dr. Williams said he had seen enough. It was not any better from the last EMG. The next step in treatment was IVIG infusions. Essentially they are antibodies harvested from donors, and the idea is that the antibodies go into the bloodstream and other antibodies destroy them instead of my body. This is a procedure that needs to be approved by insurance, at a cost of around $9,000 per infusion.

In the second week of August 2014, I started the IVIG infusions. I would have five days of infusions. Overall, everything went well. I was still on 60 milligrams of prednisone, and the plan was to start tapering off soon. One side effect of the IVIG is blood clots.

The week after infusion, our family headed to Hilton Head, South Carolina, for a vacation. It was on the ride there that I noticed a lot of swelling. During our five-day vacation, something alerted me to another issue—the swelling didn't go down as much. After returning home, I then took a flight to Texas to visit my parents. The swelling noticeably increased there, and during the flight. Since I had received a lot of blood product, maybe the fluid given with the infusions was the culprit.

My parents noticed the swelling too. As all families do when facing medical issues, we made our own diagnosis: it was just the fluid. I returned home, went back to work, and made the monthly follow-up with Dr. Williams. After a month on the IVIG, I can say that my leg strength came back, so I assumed this was working. This was good news. I was able to go up stairs and down stairs better. I communicated this to Dr. Williams. He was glad to hear it, but then I asked about my legs. He looked at them, called the nurse in, and ordered an ultrasound "stat." In an hour, I was diagnosed with a DVT (Deep Vein Thrombosis) in both legs, two in the right and one in the left. Here we go again. More questions.

Another Road

Dr. Williams had immediately put me on a blood thinner. I went to see a vascular doctor the next week, and he confirmed and detailed the diagnosis. I was going to be watched for the next six months for changes in the DVT. To make a long story short, the blood clots didn't change. During this time, Dr. Williams began to taper me off the prednisone. It was awful. After my last dose, the following week brought fatigue, some vomiting, and knots in my stomach. I was so tired and weak and felt just plain bad.

I decided that I should see an endocrinologist after seeing that prednisone can mess with the endocrine system. Well, it sure did. I had a high glucose reading, high end of A1C (historic blood sugar levels) test, and now an oddly functioning thyroid. I was diagnosed with hypothyroidism. By then I was already on blood thinner, and now I am taking a medication to help boost the thyroid. So I was getting old, right?

Entering the Christmas season of 2014, I was having some tingling in my feet, a blood clot, hypothyroidism, and a developing issue with my toenail. The nail was ingrown and looked to be digging into the skin. So I did some homemade clipping to solve the problem. Due to the pain in my bones from prednisone, I thought, I was taking two ibuprofen a day. Then came 2015, a year that I will never forget.

The Downhill Slide

I started out the year somewhat with the idea it was going to be a good one. Dr. Williams had started back with the IVIG infusions. I had started to notice some weakness again in my legs. We went with a smaller dose of two days. This occurred in January, March, April, and June. Each time I noticed no difference and didn't feel a bit better.

The second week of January, my toe had become so painful that I went to the doctor, who took the toenail off. He diagnosed a staph infection as well. Antibiotics were the course of action. The weekend to come brought about the beginning of the fast slide to near death.

I came home from church that Sunday afternoon. All of the sudden, I noticed an unusual pain in my upper abdomen. I'd had indigestion before, yet this didn't seem that way. It was pain going to my back. I ate a sandwich, which proved not to help. My concern was where the pain was. My thought was of blood clots possibly moving to my lungs or heart. I came out of the bedroom to tell my wife I was going to the ER. On arriving at the ER, I explained I might have a pulmonary embolism. They reacted quickly. I had tests and X-rays, but there was no embolism. The pain began to get worse. After a CT, ultrasound, labs, and no telling what else, I still had no answers. I could sit still, but I was dry heaving and in pain I don't care to ever see again.

I went home about 9:00 p.m. I could not lie down long before I was in the fetal position on the floor again. At 3:00 a.m., my wife took me to a different ER. More tests, a little more details research, two rounds of pain meds, and I was still in pain. The doctor was guessing an ulcer or something to do with the stomach. I was able to get in to see a GI doctor two days later. She gave me some different meds, which helped, and the next day, I had an endoscopy. Her diagnosis was gastritis.

I lost ten pounds during this time, which was about five days. It was now February 2015. We were moving right along, right? March and April were normal, I suppose. I weighed 215 at the start of January, and now I was around 200. My appetite was the same, but I was losing weight. I assumed it was from the bout of gastritis.

By then, I'd had gastritis, DVT, high glucose, a staph infection in the toe, a toenail removed, and weight loss. It was in April 2015 that I started to notice some serious changes. My weight was still at 200. The weight I lost from the gastritis battle in January had not recovered. Dr. Williams continued with the IVIG treatments, but nothing was better.

I went back to the gastric doctor to address my concerns with weight loss. She recommended a colonoscopy. Great, I thought. Since there was no obvious reason for my weight loss, I assumed this would help get some answers. The colonoscopy result was normal. She said there were no signs of anything, all looked well, and she took some biopsy to send off, but nothing ever came back abnormal.

In July of 2015, we took a trip to Colorado, where we planned to join my parents. When we arrived in Denver, my parents were already there. They almost fainted because of how skinny and purple looking I was. During this trip, I stayed lethargic most of the time. Sitting in our resort room one evening, my parents and wife suggested I call Johns Hopkins for a second opinion. I had nothing to lose. In late July, weighing in at 180 pounds, with a sunk-in face, weak, tripping, and tired, I knew it was time to do something else.

The Smoking Gun

On August 28, 2015, I took a flight to Baltimore, Maryland, for a second opinion with Johns Hopkins neurologist Dr. Khoshnoodi. The visit went well, and he agreed with the current diagnosis, but he wanted more blood work and an EMG (again). The afternoon was spent completing these tests. Around 6:00 p.m., I called Uber and went back to the hotel for pizza and wings.

My flight back to Atlanta was on Saturday, August 29. That following Wednesday, as I was sitting in a driveway and making a UPS delivery, the phone rang. It was Dr. Khoshnoodi calling. These are his remarks as best I can remember, because they are hard to forget: "Mr. Horton, I agree with your diagnosis of CIPD, the EMG showed demyelination of the nerves, but I did another blood test called a VEGF test, and it was elevated."

"Okay," I replied.

He then uttered the words I'll never forget: "I think you may have POEMS syndrome, and you need to see a hematologist soon."

I said, "How elevated was it?"

He replied, "Normal is 30 to 88, and yours was 962." I was stunned and shocked, yet it made sense. I drove off from that driveway that Wednesday morning, not knowing my life was about to change.

The Diagnosis

Dealing with a medical diagnosis is a big battle for anyone. At the time I'm writing this book, I have friends who are dealing with medical issues that have greatly affected their lives. One friend is in a particularly hard fight against an aggressive cancer. Proverbs 27:1 says, *"Do not boast about tomorrow, for you do not know what a day may bring,"* and that defines how I now live my life. We are simply not guaranteed another second beyond what we already have. Life changes in a moment's notice. Just the other night, after midnight, my wife's phone rang, and our hearts sank, but it was the wrong number. We don't know what the next doctor's appointment will bring. This is not a gloomy outlook, it is a reality. This is life, and we are like a vapor or mist as James 4:14 defines, *"You do not know what tomorrow will bring. What is your life? For you are a mist that appears for a little time and then vanishes."*

I have noticed people often deal with trivia on a daily basis.

Too many silly things occupy our lives. Sometimes it takes a serious diagnosis to set things in order. However, a diagnosis is not always a sign you are not living as you should. Many times, such a diagnosis simply refines our focus. There is not a single promise in the Scriptures to us for an "easy" life here on this earth. Job 14:1 says, *"Man who is born of a woman is few of days and full of trouble."* That is life here, not the eternal life we have through Christ. Keeping this truth in mind helps me to know that the diagnosis I received was a part of life, but it's not eternal life.

None of us are going to live forever. We may think we are at a young age, because the end of life never comes to mind. As I struggled through my pre-diagnosis health issues, I felt as if the end was nearing. I just was not getting any better in spite of the doctor visits and medications I was getting. Life is always going to be full of decisions, trials, rough patches, and difficult hills to climb. Yes, there are days that life is like being at the beach, but even there in what seems to be a perfect place lie danger, riptides, and jellyfish. Enjoy each moment that the Lord gives you. Don't fret over the little things that take your joy.

The Mayo Clinic

I had always heard about the Mayo Clinic. Though the grapevine, I knew it was a place that people went to get the help they could not find anywhere else. On September 11, 2015, I sat at the dining room table, going over the possible diagnosis of POEMS from my Johns Hopkins visit. I spoke with the neurologist at Johns Hopkins, and in turn, he spoke to the hematology department at Johns Hopkins. I called, expressed the urgency of what had been discovered, and learned the earliest appointment I could get to see the hematologist was in April of 2017. I was devastated. With my hands buried in my face on the dining room table, I cried out, "Lord, you have to do something." It was not a prayer, it was a plea. No asking God for something, I just cried out in desperation.

I was not mad at God by any means, but I knew he was the only one that could help now. Six to eight months to see a doctor about a deadly plasma cell disorder? No, God had to intervene. Psalms 3:4 says, *"I cried aloud to the LORD, and he answered me from his holy hill."* Psalms 18:6 says, *"In my distress I called upon the LORD; to my God I cried for help."* In my own desperate moment, I made a cry to the Lord for intervention. Call it a prayer or whatever, but he's my father, and I needed help.

I Googled the Mayo Clinic for locations. It was 1:10 p.m. on a Friday. My thoughts were not very positive. My wife came into the dining room, and I looked at her and said, "Great, I have found out I have a deadly disease, and now I'm going to die because I can't get in to the doctor." Friends, that was exactly how I felt. I felt as if I were alone at sea with only a small life raft amid fifteen-foot waves. I felt helpless.

I looked at the Mayo Clinic website, plugged in the possible diagnosis of POEMS, and up came some of the most encouraging news I had seen. The Mayo was a leading researcher

19

for the disorder. Many cases had been treated over the past few years, although the disease was still not common. Now all I needed was someone to see me. I began to dial the number in hopes of a miracle.

My explanation to the one who answered the appointment line was frank, quick, and somewhat desperate. I explained what the doctor at Johns Hopkins had suspected. I told her of the rarity of my diagnosis and how I needed to see a hematologist. I didn't know if she sensed my desperation, but she put me on hold for around five minutes. She came back on the line, around two o'clock, and said, "Let me call you back, Mr. Horton." I said, "Uh, okay."

As I sat there thinking of the time frame that Friday, and of the desperation of my diagnosis, I called my dad to tell him the current situation. My parents said they would be going to the next appointment with me, no matter where it was. I don't recall the totality of how I felt that Friday afternoon, but it seemed as if I was at a standstill, dying, I thought. I am not sure what I did after that, possibly more Internet research about POEMS syndrome.

At 4:45 p.m., my phone rang. I saw the number, and it was the area code for the Mayo Clinic. I answered nervously.

The lady on the end of the line said, "I have spoken with the doctors in the hematology department, and two of them want to see you soon." Then she said, "But the soonest I have is the twenty-fourth."

I said, "The twenty-fourth of what?"

"September," she replied.

I believe I shouted. That was only thirteen days away, and it sure beat seven months. My records would be sent as soon as possible, and I ended the conversation with joy. Now, I might get some help.

The Trip We Had Been Waiting For

Everyone anticipates a vacation they have planned for a while. The days get longer as the final moment approaches. For me, it was a long ten days. At that point, I was still working, albeit with difficulty. My days were long, long, and very long. My normal workday was around ten hours, but compounded by physical conditions, pain, and weakness, it seemed much longer. I dreaded getting into my truck, getting out, and moving packages around. Hills were like mountains, and long driveways and high steps all seemed treacherous.

My mom and dad had specifically said they would be with us for this doctor trip. My dad, to this day, still says he should have gone with me to Johns Hopkins. I tell him repeatedly that it is fine, but he still worries. By mid-evening, my parents had the tickets to Atlanta via Southwest Airlines, and our plans were to pick them up at the airport and then head south via I-75 to Jacksonville.

Knowing this day was coming was hugely welcome in my life. I knew one of two things would be the outcome. Either I would have the disease that I was suspected of having or it would be something else, far worse, far more unimaginable.

We went south on a journey of hope. We had a good time on the trip—a family trip that was anything but a vacation. My mother had all the entertainment lined up, including cards, games, and fun activities for the kids. Her job was to be the babysitter while my dad, wife, and I were at the doctor. She did a good job.

The Office Visit

September 24 finally came. The Mayo Clinic was so efficient. We arrived around nine o'clock for the check-in. I was amazed at the efficiency of even the check-in process. We went from one station to another, never waiting long at all. The first stop was for lab work at 9:45. We checked in to the lab area, waited five to ten minutes, and I was off.

We had about two hours between labs and the doctor's appointment, which was at 11:45 a.m. We decided to get a bite to eat at the cafeteria. At 11:15 a.m., I checked the Mayo Clinic app I had downloaded on my iPhone. There was a button for "labs," so I looked at it, and most of my results were already back. I was amazed. The entire clinic was patient oriented. It was all about you, the patient, and the disease. I felt as if I was being cared about at every step of the process.

Next came checking in to see the doctor, the moment we had been praying for. As I sat there about to go in, my heart was full. I prayed for answers, help, and for God to be kind to me. I still was apprehensive as my doubts rose up. I knew I was sick, and I knew it was getting bad. I let the doubts overtake my faith.

I know now those lack-of-faith moments were overtaken by a sovereign God who works no matter the amount of faith I have or not. He is faithful when we are not.

Dr. Swaika came in, and from the very onset, he was detailed, helpful, hopeful, and dedicated. He had obtained my pile of medical records from the past year or so of different medical issues, but the one that interested him most was the VEGF (Vascular endothelial growth factor) test. This particular test looks for anti-bodies in overbalance in the blood. In fact, as he was looking through the results, he came to that one and his eyes became enlarged at the result. I believe he was somewhat stunned by the results of this test.

A thorough examination followed, with details of all the symptoms and problems that I was having. Looking at me, he said, "We have to do our tests, but it seems to me that you may very likely have POEMS." He mentioned that he was going to discuss this with another doctor, as that is the standard at the Mayo, and he said it would be twenty to thirty minutes. We waited.

I met with Dr. Swaika and Dr. Ailawadhi, who was a leading doctor in treating this disease. I was his third POEMS case in 2015. Their straightforward yet compassionate care was incredible. Dr. Ailawadhi explained the timeline for treating the disease if indeed it was POEMS. I was to undergo a battery of tests, a bone scan, an ultrasound, and a twenty-four-hour urine test. We had set aside several days for the visit, so we stayed at the Mayo for three days. We made the best of our time by enjoying some tours and visiting the oldest city in America, St. Augustine. I also had time to think about the future.

Before we left, the doctors laid out the plan—four to six months of oral chemotherapy, then a stem cell transplant. I didn't really know what to think but why me? At the same time, I found myself thinking, the Lord has brought me to the right place. As we left, a follow-up appointment was already scheduled for October 7, 2015. That seemed as if it were too many days away, only ten, but I knew the disease was progressing. Every day seemed long and painful.

The Tests And The Reason

We left the office around 12:45 p.m. that day. I think of Psalms 20:1: *"May the Lord answer you in the day of trouble! May the name of the God of Jacob protect you."* I was troubled, and to see the hand of God move was and still is fascinating. Dr. Swaika said he needed a bone scan, an ultrasound, more blood labs, and a twenty-four-hour urine test. He said it usually took a couple of days to schedule the bone scan and ultrasound. We could start the test for the twenty-four-hour urine immediately. We were totally prepared to stay or even come back to get an answer. As we left his office, before we could get out of the waiting room, he came out with a schedule. I was to be at the ultrasound center on the sixth floor at 2:15 p.m. and for a bone scan on the seventh floor at 3:45 p.m. that very day!

Say what you will about faith. I had no faith these tests would be done that day, but the Lord who is faithful did. He worked through a system of men to coordinate tests to be done the same day. *"May the Lord answer you in the day of trouble"* is as real today as it ever was. My dad and I were stunned. In fact, we still talk about how quickly things transpired. Psalms 20:7 says, *"Some trust in chariots and some in horses; but we trust in the name of the Lord our God."*

Speaking frankly, it is the Lord who moves upon people, whether they are believers or not. He moved through the appointment system, the testing system, and the other details during this season of my life. I don't doubt that.

Saturday rolled around, and we prepared to make our way back to Atlanta. After two days at the Mayo, now we waited. We had some good, thoughtful discussions on the way home, and most of all, we were encouraged that we might have some answers.

POEMS

On October 7, 2015, my wife, our two youngest kids, and I made our way back to the Mayo Clinic. It was a Wednesday, and I continued to work at UPS during that time. I worked two days that week, and I remember that on Tuesday, October 6, I was really hurting. It seemed as if I was starting to shut down.

We loaded up the family van around five o'clock that morning for a 2:00 p.m. appointment. Arriving at the Mayo, being checked in, and waiting on Dr. Swaika to come in, I honestly didn't know what to think. After being in the room for only a few minutes, the doctor came in and said, "There's no doubt you have POEMS." It was a relief to have a diagnosis, but I didn't know what to think at the same time. Good, but now what?

We heard the plan for how we would treat the disease. Dr. Ailawadhi, who has been a leading expert in the treatment of POEMS, came in. Very kindly, he explained the timeline for treating the disease—four to six month of oral chemotherapy and steroid treatment, then a stem cell transplant. The goal was to get the disease under control, then wipe it out.

One of the leading strategies in treating POEMS is to gain control of it. This allows the patient to regain some ground lost to the disease, all in preparation for the stem cell transplant. At the time of diagnosis, I was unhealthy looking and weighed 178 pounds. My face was sunk in, my skin was a purple-looking color, and I could walk only with great difficulty. The doctors at Mayo determined the progress of treatment by both my lab work and my physical condition.

POEMS is a rare, multi-symptomatic disorder. I believe many people in the world die because disorders or diseases are not properly diagnosed. Dying may not be because of lack of quality health care, but these diseases are not well known. This was the case with POEMS. I met with my neurologist at Emory to get his thoughts. He knew about POEMS and had been involved in researching it at one time, but still he was not familiar enough with it. However, he was not offended at our suggestion but was encouraged, and he set off to call the hematologist I was seeing in Atlanta.

I made an appointment with that hematologist, expecting an answer to POEMS, but he thought the syndrome was a "myth." In fact, it appeared to me that he had not done any research of the disease prior to our visit. All he wanted to do was schedule another bone marrow extraction. I ran out as fast as I could.

My visit to the Mayo Clinic was to confirm the diagnosis of my having POEMS syndrome based on Johns Hopkins's findings. The doctors at the Mayo Clinic were very detailed. Given the facts already presented, confirmation was the key. No specific case definition exists for POEMS syndrome; however, most authorities agree that patients with POEMS syndrome should have three or more of the five markers. Some doctors have proposed that the presence of two major criteria, including a monoclonal plasma-proliferative disorder and polyneuropathy, in addition to the existence of one minor criterion, is sufficient for diagnosis. It seemed that I had more criteria than needed when I was diagnosed.

In addition to that, I factored in the VEGF test, which was highly elevated at 962, supposed to be maximum 88, and I was hitting on all cylinders. One can look at the Internet to find out mounds of information regarding POEMS. Opinions abound, research abounds, and real life stories differ. The fact is my doctors had confirmed the diagnosis, and by God's grace the treatment began.

So there we were, knowing exactly what was the cause of my health decline. Now what? I gave consideration again to

Romans 8:28: *"And we know that for those who love God all things work together for good, for those who are called according to his purpose."* I have quoted that all my Christian life, but learning it seems to be the more difficult process. How does all this work out? How can an illness work for the good? Often we don't see the end results, but God does. We press on knowing that we have hope beyond this life. I left the doctor's office that day with energy I cannot explain, knowing that if the Lord wills, he will heal. I had peace that God is sovereign.

PREPARATION AND PROVIDENCE

On October 7, 2015, I was diagnosed with POEMS syndrome. As I was sitting in the doctor's office that afternoon, the plan was laid out. My diagnosis was confirmed with overwhelming evidence. I was to start a Revlimid and Dexamethasone combination. The Revlimid is a 25-milligram chemotherapy pill, which I would take for twenty-one days and then be off seven. I was to take 40 milligrams of Dexamethasone, a steroid, once a week. Every thirty days, I was to see the doctor to monitor my progress.

On October 10, 2015, the medicine arrived at my house. It was a big day for me. I was at home alone awaiting the arrival of the drugs while my wife and family were gone to a family reunion. The medicine arrived, but I hesitated taking it until about an hour before bedtime. It was suggested that I pick a time and stick to it. At this point in the disease, I weighed about 177 pounds. I normally weighed about 215. I looked bad, really bad. My face was sunk in, my skin was discolored, I could barely walk, and it hurt to turn over in bed. I could go on, but you get my drift.

My wife arrived home around seven o'clock. Rhonda made some phone calls to a friend who has had the disease, and they had a good hour-long conversation and prayer. Then at 9:00 p.m., I took the pill. Game on. It was a day I won't forget. I still remember the shirt I had on, the bear shirt I had bought in Colorado. I waited now for the effects of the pill.

I knew this course was my preparation for the stem cell or bone marrow transplant (BMT). The transplant process had been explained briefly to us. We knew it would require a hospital stay of several weeks, and we would need to be close by for doctor visits and lab work. The drive time from our house to the Mayo Clinic in Jacksonville, Florida, was six and a half hours. We had it down pat by now. We knew where to stop and fuel, eat, and all the rest areas. What lay before us, even though it was months away, was the transplant. We had a lot of logistical issues, four kids, and a myriad of things to sort out.

Emory Or Mayo

It wasn't until the December visit to the doctor that we were told we should consider getting consults at both the Mayo Clinic and Emory University Hospital for the bone marrow transplant (BMT). These things took time and planning. Having a BMT was not like having a standard medical procedure. It was a big deal. It was not just a big deal, it was a life-saving deal. It was like getting a new birthday.

Before us were two choices. The doctors at Mayo had no issue with doing the BMT near our home at Emory in Atlanta. Emory was an hour away from our home. Logistically, having it done there would be easier. On the way home from Florida, on December 8, 2015, I made the call to the BMT office at Emory. I requested a meeting with the doctor that was recommended by Mayo, which was familiar with my disease. The coordinator received all the necessary information from me and said she would contact Mayo, have records sent, and set the appointment. All was set, and things were moving nicely.

A few days before Christmas, while visiting my parents in Texas, I called Emory again to check on the status of the appointment. I had no luck in having my phone calls returned. It seemed there was great difficulty in getting an appointment. I was a planner by nature, and not having a plan really made me not tick too well. I knew that if I were to move forward with the transplant, upon finishing the last round of oral chemo, I had to have things in order. I wanted the transplant to take place at Emory, and I didn't want to burden my family with a few months away from home in Florida, although Florida was nice in the spring.

I sent an email to my doctor at the Mayo Clinic on December 18, 2015. On December 22, my app for the Mayo Clinic sent me an alert saying I had an appointment with the BMT team on January 26, 2016. My stomach sank, and I knew this thing was moving forward. The monthly doctor visit was on

January 5, 2016. I was in the fourth cycle of my oral chemo treatment. As we prepared for the monthly visit, I knew I had to make some decisions soon.

One of the most important decisions to make was where to have treatment. We had two options before us, one an hour away and the other six hours away. If you are considering similar options, the obvious choice doesn't always work the best. My wife was leaning heavily toward Emory, and I understood why. I was leaning heavily toward Mayo. I was comfortable there, the doctors worked together, and the hospital doctors were all in the same place. These were difficult decisions that had to be weighed. I learned that the more difficult choice, the harder and less logistical choice, might be the best.

On January 5, 2016, we met with my hematologist. He asked, "Have you made an appointment with Emory?" We had finally made an appointment for February 5, 2016. It was not even with the BMT team. We told him we had an appointment with Mayo's BMT team on January 26. He was excited. He said, "Wherever you go, do it quick." I knew then that we were at the right place. The labs showed the VEGF level and other blood labs to be in the right range for transplant. My doctor was pleased with physical improvements, along with my lab work. Both showed the disease was in regression, and it was time to move forward with the transplant. It wouldn't be long now.

The Big Decision

There was one thing we could say about the process at the

Mayo, that everything was in sync and seemed to be in perfect working order. Everyone seemed to be on top of their game, all the time. The day arrived for us to leave for the Mayo BMT meeting. The meeting began with a doctor we had not previously met. He was a part of the entire hematology/oncology team at Mayo. He explained in detail the process of the stem cell transplant. The labs all looked good, as they pointed toward remission of the disease. Then he said, "I am going to go review this with Dr. Roy (the head of the BMT team) to see if he wants to continue another cycle of oral chemo." When he left the room, I felt devastated, because I did not want to continue on that, I wanted to get the transplant over with. We knew we were meeting with the doctor at Emory a week after this appointment, so we were comfortable with whoever was able to do it the quickest. Whoever we felt the most comfortable with, that's where we would go.

Dr. Roy came in with his team of nurses. He looked at us and said, "I believe you're ready for the transplant." Wow, relief and fear appeared at the same time. I don't know if you have ever faced those two at once, but it was stunning. He asked how long we would be staying in town. It was Tuesday, and we had planned on leaving Wednesday. He ordered a CT scan, an ultrasound, and more labs. Those were to be done on Tuesday and Wednesday. We assumed that once results from these came in, the BMT team would give us a date for transplant. We would talk with Emory and learn their pace for a transplant. Little did we know that the snowball had begun to roll, and it would roll very quickly.

We weighed our options. On the way to pick up some snacks and get some lunch, as we sat down to eat, I checked my Mayo app on my iPhone. It had twenty-seven appointments scheduled beginning on February 6, 2016—the day after the scheduled Emory appointment. After speaking with the nurse coordinator, we learned that the appointments were for an EKG, echochardiogram, lung test, blood work, and a meeting with the nurse BMT coordinator. Based on this information, Mayo was ready to start the pre-transplant workup, stem cell preparation for harvesting and transplant day, on February 23. We were stunned at the fast-paced movement of this process. We had much to do.

The next week, I made the trip back to the Mayo with two of my kids, giving my wife a break from travel. She had been such a great help. I was feeling really well since my diagnosis a few months earlier. Before the trip, we sat around the dining room table and she said, "Maybe the Mayo is the best place for this." After seeing the efficient workings of the hospital, doctors, and staff, it seemed to be the most comfortable place to do this. However, what lay ahead was a task. Where would we stay? How would we do this?

Finding A Place To Stay

When the rubber meets the road, a man will do whatever is necessary to survive. That is, to survive in this life. I know my life is not my own, it is God's. Yet through his divine favor, I live. God always provides. He never fails, not one single time. The providential hand of God is in the details of life. We often think of God as doing only the big things, yet he is real in even the very smallest areas of our life. For me, it was finding a place to stay.

This would make the seventh trip to Jacksonville. In the midst of trials, I have often tried to make the best of them. In other words, the trial is painful and hard, but if it is possible, then make the best of it. So I tried. I took my second and fourth children with me, my sixteen-year-old daughter and seven-year-old son. Those two are just alike; he loves his big sister, and she cherishes him. It would not be a fun trip full of free time because we would be busy for most of the time. After arriving Tuesday afternoon, we had some time to settle in. The schedule included labs, lung tests, heart tests, ultrasounds, and other meetings with the team to determine the readiness of my body for the transplant. All of this was routine to me, but what was not routine was being able to find accommodations. That seemed to be the biggest obstacle, trying to logistically plan for six to eight weeks in Florida, with at least two adults to care for me after transplant.

We were told to plan for two months in Florida. We needed to be near the clinic after hospital dismissal so I could have labs twice a week. So we set the plan in order. Arriving back in Florida on February 6, we were to be there through February 8. This visit consisted of the preliminary procedures prior to staying for the transplant. I had several tests, a CT scan, ultrasounds, lung tests, and meetings with a social worker, psychologist, and BMT team again.

When someone is having medical treatment, a lot of logistics are involved. Even close to home, a person needs transportation, labs, and help for getting day-to-day things done. When you are having treatment hours away from home, the challenges grow. Something I am learning is that God orchestrates things in order to accomplish his purpose, and yes, that's even in the details of finding accommodations, doctors, and moving upon the hearts of those approving tests with the insurance company. I had a challenge before me to find a place that week, because the next week, beginning February 11, 2016, I would be there for pre-transplant workup and then the transplant. Time was critical.

Options, Price, And Where To Stay

I am no dummy when it comes to understanding the value of a dollar. I don't have enough dollars to throw around without considering where they go. For many people seeking medical treatment, having the funds for accommodations is the biggest issue. Frankly, accommodations are not cheap. Discounts are available through hospital arrangements, but even then, it can still be very expensive. I began to search the Internet, social media, and any other means I could find. The first option was the extended-stay hotels. They had a full kitchen, two beds, and one bath. The other option I researched, even using real estate agents, was short-term leasing of a house. The truth is I never felt comfortable with the extended-stay option. There was simply not enough room for five people. The only comfortable option in such a hotel would be to rent two rooms, and the cost began to add up.

I contacted real estate agents to see about renting a house. Short-term rentals seemed a viable option for Florida in the spring. It was. The problem was that the time we needed the rental was springtime, February and March. A phenomenon that happens in Florida each spring is called spring break. The cost of house rentals is high, plus inventory is low. Strike two. Three strikes and you're out in baseball, but this was not baseball.

I found a website that offered short-term apartment rentals. I called to find out availability, and of course there was none. I spent some time discussing the options with the manager. These places came fully furnished and with cable, Wi-Fi, a mailbox, access to the business office, a pool, a common area with shuffleboard, coffee, and much more. It was a gated property as well. I felt this would be so nice since my wife and kids would be by themselves a lot. The bottom line? Availability, price, and convenience were really hard to come by.

On Friday, we left the Mayo Clinic after a meeting with the nutritionist. Headed west on the 202, I felt a little nervous. A lot needed to come together for this. It was February 5, my dad was flying to Atlanta on February 11, and we were headed to Jacksonville that day for pre-transplant workup, stem cell collection, and port surgery starting February 12. Time was closing in.

On the 202 highway, halfway to I-95 for our trip home, the phone rang. It was Denise, the manager at the Corporate Suite Shoppe. She said, "You're not going to believe this, Brad. I had someone move out today, first floor, two bedrooms in a luxury apartment, and it will be ready for you on the eleventh." I almost drove off the road. Now what she meant by "luxury" was a gated apartment with security and a nice, comfortable place for my family to stay and for me to recover after the transplant. It was fully furnished, all utilities were included, and all we needed was the key. I said we would take it.

There you have it, God moving upon people to help me. For many of you considering the transplant away from home, the accommodations are important. The apartment rental for us for each month was $2,500. That was a lot for a man like me. In fact, I felt it was too much. But considering the options and numbers, here is what I came up with.

Where To Stay, Why To Stay There, And Comfort

The place where you stay during recovery matters very much, to the family and to you. Let me say this as a matter of serious consideration. Paying more for a nice, comfortable place, if possible, is worth it. Let me be transparent: you'll need some privacy. If you're having trouble with sickness, having a private bathroom is essential. In a hotel room, this would not be possible. If that's all you have, then so be it. However, if options are available, this is a major criteria. You will want to just rest and be alone many times. It was great to have a bedroom where

I could shut the door and be by myself when I wasn't feeling well. Others could go on about their business without fear of bothering me or seeing me not feel well. It turned my parents' stomachs to see me feeling bad. My dad would ask many times what he could do, knowing he could do nothing. If my parents could have helped, they would have.

When I considered the extended-stay hotels, which are a good option if needed, the room came with a double or queen bed (two of them) and a full kitchen. Again, there would be no privacy, and with caregivers joining us as well, there would not have been enough room for everyone, so two rooms would have been required. The cost for a thirty-day stay at the places I checked was $1,890. So I considered what I was getting with the extended-stay hotel and the apartment and made my decision. Yes, I would pay $500 more. However, I had two bedrooms, two baths, a pool, a common area, all utilities paid, and the great part was that during the two-month stay, we met neighbors we still have contact with.

I am not foolish and know that neither of those options is cheap. You will be amazed at what you can do with the Lord's help in times of crisis and how he will provide in order to sustain you. We were blessed to have this option before us. It made the recovery after I was released from the hospital easier, it was comfortable for my family to stay there while I recovered, and it was almost a second home to us by the time we left. I am grateful for the good hand of the Lord upon us to provide.

THE HOSPITAL STAY

It began February 22, 2016. This was the day of my admission to the Mayo Clinic in Jacksonville, Florida, for the stem cell transplant. The process consisted of harvesting my own stem cells a week before, then high-dose chemotherapy, and the following day, transplanting the stem cells back into my body.

A funny thing about life is that it will end at some point. I was brought face to face with this truth even though I know that someday, my life will end. In fact, we are dying, and unless the Lord returns, we will all face the hand of death. The hopeful truth is that for the believer, the Lord's return is the fulfillment of a promise that you will be with God. We see this in 2 Corinthians 5:8: *"Yes, we are of good courage, and we would rather be away from the body and at home with the Lord."* I thought often of this because if not treated, I would be at home with God sooner rather than later. What if something went wrong and I didn't make it through the transplant? Well, hello, temporary life. I knew what this meant.

Knowing that, I found that a lot of emotions and thoughts transpired in those fifteen days in the hospital. One of the most important things I have learned in my life is to be honest about reality. Don't sugarcoat anything to make it more plausible. Just lay it out straight. Preachers of the gospel who stand in the pulpit each week need to grasp that we too struggle with life issues. We also are not exempt from sickness, temptations, struggles, emotional battles, depression, and weak spiritual moments. Friends, if you want to get depressed or struggle to be "happy," then confine yourself to a hospital room for fifteen days.

Day One

On February 22, 2016, Rhonda and I entered the Mayo Clinic Hospital at 05:30. It looked as if I was going to the airport. I had my rolling luggage packed with my laptop, phone, books, pajama shorts (I don't do pajama pants), and shirts. As we arrived, I was welcomed into Room 341. I will never forget that number. My wife was there with me as we got settled in. Nurses made their way in, checked all the information, and waited on the day shift staff to be briefed. Somewhere around 7:15 a.m., the nurses rolled in with medications and began to explain what was about to happen. You think you're tough, as I do, but you soon realize that your body, which God made, is about to be bombed. Everything God created to work—the bone marrow, the stem cells, the white and red cells—was about to be attacked. It was

41

the moment I realized that it was possible I might not come through this. Seriously, I did.

The plan was to start with premedication via my port in my chest, antibiotics, and antifungal and antinausea medicine. That was to start at 10:00 a.m. The chemo was to start at 11:00 a.m. So I waited as I looked at the bag of clear liquid that I knew was killing my cells, marrow, and possibly whatever else it came into contact with. I was placed on a heart monitor, and blood tests would be done at midnight.

One of the common side effects of this high-dose chemo is mouth sores. I am told they are very painful. Many who have had mouth sores have been on pain pumps to get through them. Over the years of conducting this type of chemo, doctors have proven that eating ice and having Popsicles will prevent the chemo from settling in the vessels of the mouth. The theory is that the ice and cold keep the vessels frozen, keeping the poison at bay. I ordered six Popsicles and three cups of ice to prevent mouth sores. It worked.

Day Two

February 24, 2016 is transplant day. It is the day that my stem cells get infused back into my body to circulate the blood to engraft into the marrow. It is my birthday, they say. I will have the immune system of a newborn once the marrow engrafts. The new transplant is to take about an hour. I'm given some premeds to ensure no reactions. It goes well. I wait to see if anything is abnormal, and thankfully it's not. I still have my appetite, so I order some lunch.

Days Three and Four

After reading about many people's experience with the AST (autologous stem cell) transplant, I was waiting for the bad days to come. I knew in my heart they would. I still felt good at this point, which was Friday and Saturday or days three and four. I felt fear because I was expecting the rough stuff to hit already. Doctors and nurses said it was coming, other patients said it was coming... so I waited.

I was feeling some fatigue. When I say "fatigue," I would later know what true fatigue is. It is not just being "worn out," it's much more than that. I knew my body was enduring something abnormal, and I praised God for these good days so far, but I knew what was coming.

Days Five, Six, and Seven

Saturday was a day that was all right, then Sunday morning brought some unpleasant stomach issues. Now that my stomach was beginning to feel the effects of chemo, they needed to see if I had a stomach bacteria. Sunday was tough, feeling as if I had been run over by a truck. I could not pinpoint one specific issue, I just felt bad all over. Monday brought some of the same issues—sickness, a blah feeling, and weakness. I felt it now.

Monday night rolled around, and I lay in the uncomfortable hospital bed. Every night around 12:30, the nurses came in to draw blood. This night was no different, and the patient care tech checked vitals every four hours. It is truly hard to rest in the hospital. That day was different, and at 5:30 a.m., the nurse came in and said, "No leaving the room for you." What that meant was that I had no immune system, and my ANC (absolute neutrophils count) was at zero. Nothing was there to protect me from infection. I was now isolated.

Days Eight through Twelve

Believe it or not, Day Eight was the day we had been waiting for, the day the ANC dropped to zero so it would begin to climb above .5 so I could leave the room again. And if the ANC was above .5 for three days, I could leave. Great! We had reached bottom, so the only place to go was up. I assumed my ANC would start to rise now. Labs were done at 12:30, a nurse came to write them on the board, and the ANC was… zero. What?

Day Eight brought some activity in my room. When my vitals were taken at 4:30 a.m., the patient care tech noted I had a fever. The nurse came in to confirm the temperature. I said I didn't feel hot, and she said, "You are at 101.9." Okay, that's hot. Tylenol was administered, and two techs came to draw blood from each arm, at the same time. IV antibiotics were started. I suppose that I began to think, "What if it is a blood infection?" Those are never good.

The fever never returned for the remainder of the stay. Of course, that was good news. My second weekend in the hospital was upon me. I expected a few days of ANC to read zero. Each morning I would look at the whiteboard, and it would read zero.

For the first time, I began to get a bit anxious.

Sunday of my second weekend in the hospital brought the first bout of vomiting. It was not a virus vomiting but a dry heaving and, well, bile coming up. I felt awful all day. Monday didn't bring much relief. I began to struggle. Honestly, I don't know of anything worse than being sick. It simply is a devastating feeling as you wait patiently for your body to recover.

The highly anticipated climb of the ANC count was on my mind. On Day+9 I was going to receive shots to boost the ANC and white count. During a stem cell transplant, whether it's autologous or donor stem cells, the stem cells have to engraft. These shots stimulate the bone marrow to produce cells. On Friday, Day+9, I received my first shot and barely saw a climb on Saturday. Sunday brought an increased count in ANC.

My hopes were now centered on getting out of the hospital. My goal was day fifteen, which would be Wednesday. Doctors were "pretty sure" I could leave. Other than some down days I had, and a fever that never returned, my handling of the transplant was good. So I began to ask the Lord for help to stay out of the danger zone because the walls were getting closer and closer to me. I was becoming quite anxious.

Days Thirteen Through Fifteen

Overall, I would say the fatigue had really begun to set in. My daily routine for years was generally waking up around 6:00 a.m. every day. I had become accustomed to this. Now I found myself sleeping until 8:00 a.m. Now that's not unusual for a lot of people, but for me it is. Not just the sleeping part but the getting out of bed. It was just a lot of work. The fatigue was something I had never felt before. Since the ANC was up, I could at least leave the room. So I began to walk around the east wing of the floor. I found that two to three trips around the floor was overwhelming. I had never felt this weak before. My legs hurt, and my muscles were suffering, it seemed. Keep in mind, I had numb feet from the disease. The numbness was there before I went to the hospital and was still persistent. So walking was always something I had to think about. Now, I was just plain tired to walk.

Being confined to a hospital room for two weeks, in the bed or the chair, had resulted in noticeable weakness. I cannot even begin to imagine the ones who have been confined to a bed for a long period of time. Muscle deteriorates fast, and I was surprised at how quickly I felt so weak.

Finally on the morning of March 8, 2016, the doctor came in and said I was ready to leave. I would have my port removed, receive discharge instructions, and be on my way out. Amen! I have to say that this was one of the happiest days of my life. Being able to leave the hospital room was overwhelming, and that in itself gave me an energy boost.

The Emotional Battles of a Hospital Stay

I am a strong man. I know that sounds a bit strange, but I am. I can do it all on my own. I don't need anyone to help me. My wife sees through that because we have been together long enough for her to know me. I entered the hospital on the twenty-third of February and had considered it a hotel stay. I had a TV, chair, couch, and bed. Room service was a phone call away. I picked up the phone, ordered what I wanted, and that was that. The menu looked really good… for a few days.

But the reality is that being a believer in Christ doesn't meant you won't struggle with depression and emotional issues. These are real issues.

First, let me say that even though you are a self-willed, strong personality, you can still have issues with depression and your emotions. No one, I mean no one, is immune. It was about day 10 when I first saw the walls closing in. The ANC was not coming up, I had been at zero for three days now, and I knew I would not be getting out until that number came up. I was fearful I would stay in the hospital longer than I had expected.

Second, let me address the fact that fear and struggles are not uncommon to Christians. We do have a source of help, the Lord. Psalms 121:1-2 says, *"I will lift up my eyes to the hills—From whence comes my help? My help comes from the LORD, Who made heaven and earth."* I know that verse because I have quoted it many times. I have often said that it is much easier to believe the verse than live it. That's not unspiritual, by the way; it is the truth.

I experienced a number of trials while staying in the hospital room. For many people, being sick is a struggle both in the body and the mind. I often think of Paul in 2 Corinthians 1:8b, *"For we were so utterly burdened beyond our strength that we despaired of life itself."* Considering that verse in context, I know that Paul is not referring to a physical sickness but persecution in general. I cannot imagine the persecution that many believers face around the world. However, many believers face the same experiences as they endure life-threatening sickness. When I see the words "despaired of life itself," I can say that I don't think I wished for life to end, but I can say that I felt I would not be able to endure it.

There are certain things that happen when you're sick. First, you don't feel like studying the Bible. It is hard to concentrate when you are feeling awful. I realized that at times during this period, I didn't pray or even feel like praying. I know there are those who say that this is the time to grow, and I don't disagree. However, the reality was that being oppressed with illness, I didn't feel like it. Did that make me less spiritual? Or less faithful? I felt as if I did not have "enough" faith.

Second, I found myself feeling as if I would never get out of the hospital. For those who have been isolated in some form, the walls begin to close in. My desire to move and be active was greatly diminished. It was warfare as I began to be bombarded with thoughts of despair.

Dismissal Day

Prior to being dismissed from the hospital, a patient must have the ANC count get over .5 for two to three days. After four days of zero counts, I became restless and feared I would have to stay longer. The bed, chair, couch, and all the amenities of room service just weren't cutting it anymore. The day before dismissal, the doctor said there was a good chance I would be dismissed the following day. My counts had risen, and I had no fevers or setbacks except for the one fever on day seven. Fears now began to arise that I would get sick, run a fever, and be held in the hospital longer. I prayed and asked the Lord for help, not only to get over this feeling of doubt but also to keep those numbers rising. "Lord, let me go home," I cried. Well, *pleaded*, anyway.

I began to walk the halls of the hospital. I did not realize how weak I had become. Not getting out of the room much had weakened my legs. Having low blood counts also added to the fatigue. It was around 9:30 a.m. when the doctor came in and said, "You can go home today. We will have you out by 1:00 p.m." I couldn't believe it. I was leaving.

After having my venous catheter removed, I was able to leave the hospital. I masked up, was wheeled out to the front, and the smell of the Florida air was tremendous. It was a warm, sunny day, and I will never forget the joy of being outside. I could not get away from Room 341 fast enough.

What I learned from the stay at the hospital is that we are all at the mercy and good graces of our God. He is faithful and trustworthy, and our feet don't hit the floor without his kind hand allowing it. I left the hospital that day praying never to see a hospital room again. To this day, I am grateful for it because it was the place of recovery, but at the same time, I hope never again to see Room 341, or any other hospital room, for that matter.

Brad L Horton

CAREGIVERS

On March 8, 2015, at 1:00 p.m., I left the Mayo Clinic Hospital. It had been a long fourteen days, and I was confined eight of those. There was a moment where I did not think I could make it another day. I was getting very restless knowing that I could recover better outside of the hospital. At least I could get some rest elsewhere. We had planned on staying nine weeks in Florida, so we rented an apartment. We were so blessed to have a short-term rental complete with a pool, a common area with some games, coffee, TV, and card table. I was confident that resting beside a pool in the Florida spring would be much better than Room 341 at the Mayo hospital.

The beautiful air of a Florida spring is something I won't forget. Walking outside to the car and feeling the sunshine hit my body was refreshing. I looked back and asked the Lord kindly for me to never see the inside of Room 341, or any other hospital room, again. I hope he honors my request.

Excitement built as we left, knowing that the recovery was official. My heart and mind wanted it to be quick, but the truth of knowing it is a day-to-day, slow process. Patience is a virtue, one that is learned by practice not preaching. I will learn it, carefully, but I will learn it. I don't have the words to describe the joy I felt as we left, the excitement of seeing my two youngest ones for the first time in three weeks. I don't remember thinking much as we left, just the feeling of God giving me a second chance.

As we made our way back to the apartment, the sun was brighter, and the sky was so clear I could hardly believe what had just happened. I do not think it takes a life-threatening illness for a man to think more clearly, but I did. I was at peace. I had confidence that God had granted me healing. Now the recovery would begin, but it wouldn't begin alone.

Emotions And Thoughts

We are emotional creatures made in the image of God. When life seems to be shortened, when there is sickness, tribulations, or trials, we get emotional. As believers, we know our hope is not in this world. We know that our eternity is with a sovereign God who knows all things. We're prepared to meet the Lord, but we have emotional family ties on earth. No one can deny such emotions.

As we began the recovery at the apartment we had rented close to the hospital, I would go back two times a week for lab work. The Lord opened up a great place for us to stay. The apartment complex was about five miles from the Mayo. It was located in an area where we were only about two miles from anything we needed. The apartment had an atmosphere of relaxation. That was the plan after the transplant, to be close by, relax, recover, and get well.

Being confined to an area and unable to do all that you may want to is tough. I sat outside, by the pool. I know, that's tough, right? I was grateful for this. However, I felt as if I would never get to where I wanted to be. There are some things that we have to learn, and one of those is patience. Being patient and letting your body find its way back to normal is not easy. My mind was working too well, I suppose, knowing that I felt better, looked better, and felt I was getting better.

Caregivers

Caregivers are an important part of the recovery process. We were given the details at our meeting with the transplant team in January. Here was our situation: We had four kids at home, ranging in age from 7 to 20. Obviously the 20-year-old and 17-year-old were well capable of managing for a time without us. We had school to complete (we homeschooled), which made the process easier. We were six hours away from home. What if one of the kids got sick? What if my wife got sick? Having a transplant is more than just something that happens to you. It also involves the lives of other people.

In January of 2016, I called my mother on the way home from Florida. I explained the plan for the pre-transplant process, the dates, and what events were to follow. I then asked her if she would be willing to come stay with us in Florida during the transplant and recovery. She replied, "I will be there throughout the whole process."

My Parents And A Backstory

My mother and dad are two unique people. I am an only child, so that makes things a little easier, I suppose. My mom retired in June of 2015. My dad is retired but drives a school bus to keep him busy. They love to travel. Sometimes they just pack up and go at a moment's notice. Besides this, they have a lifestyle they enjoy, friends who like to gather, and they are heavily involved in the local VFW (Veterans of Foreign Wars).

My mother never thought twice about putting all that on hold to come help with the kids, keep them occupied, and play cards with them while I recovered. I asked her to come with my wife and me to meet with the transplant team in January 2016. This would give her the opportunity to meet the doctors, hear the plan, and know what the process would be. After meeting with the team, I began to see appointments in the app for the Mayo. I knew that we were moving forward. We had opportunity to lay out the plans.

Knowing these details, we were able to make a plan. My mother is a planner, and she began the details of her part. However, given all the room we had available, we assured my dad that we were fine. He did play a part, though. He was to be the set-up man. Roughly ten to twelve days before the scheduled start of transplant, there was to be blood work, stem cell harvesting, and a venous catheter put into my chest. We would also be in Florida for about eight to ten weeks. Preparations needed to be made, and we needed to gather supplies for the apartment—food, coat hangers, laundry baskets, things we don't realize we need when we are at home.

The Set-Up Man

The set-up man was in charge of all this. We made the plan. My dad would arrive at the airport in Atlanta on Wednesday, February 11. I would pick him up, and we would head south to Jacksonville. I still remember the excitement of a road trip with my dad. It would be fun. Even though I knew what the purpose was, I was a little intimidated by it. Our schedule was running smooth. We arrived in Jacksonville around 6:45 p.m., located the apartment, got the key out of the lock box, and were amazed at the quality of the complex. We were relieved. The Lord had given me peace about this. It felt like home.

On Thursday, February 12, we met with the transplant team, and in the afternoon, we started injections to boost my white blood cell count. We made a few trips to the Mayo each day. My dad hopped into the driver's seat each time, doing his caregiving work. Thursday through Sunday were mostly uneventful. The shots to boost my white count made me feel as though I was coming down with a cold and upset my stomach some, but it was nothing worrisome.

Monday, my dad had me at the hospital at 6:45 a.m. to

have a port put into my chest. This was to make blood draws and to deliver chemo, stem cells, and medication. It went as well as could be expected. I was sore and tired from the procedure, but we were home by 11:00 a.m. After lunch, I lay down for a nap.

Waking up around 1:30 p.m., I noticed blood running down my stomach. I could tell it was coming from the port. I asked my dad to look at it, and he jumped into action and said, "We have to go to the hospital now."

"Okay," I replied. I made a call to the doctor as we were on the way and was whisked back into the staging area for these procedures. All was well. The port was just leaking a bit, and it was patched up and resulted in no other problems. The point is, that's what caregivers are for. He was there for me. He took over, got me to the hospital, and cared. End of story.

My dad's flight was leaving Wednesday, February 17. The set-up man had done his job. He prepared the apartment with the necessary things for us. He took me to the doctors every day, cooked supper, and most of all, we enjoyed time in the Florida weather. My final day of stem cell harvest was the day he was to return to Dallas. We were there at 6:30 a.m., finished by 11:45 a.m., and off to the airport for his 2:00 p.m. flight. As I left the airport, I thought to myself, "I should be taking care of him, but instead he was taking care of me." It is amazing that the Lord had allowed my parents to be in good health at this time. God knew I would be in this health crisis all along. I didn't.

My wife and three of my four kids were arriving the

evening I took dad to the airport. This was going to be a commitment on their part. Life was being put on hold in Georgia for me. Life would go on as somewhat normal, but it would be in Florida. School was still to be conducted, but there would also be me to care for. My wife is a trouper and a super mom, but schooling, working from home, and now a husband who was enduring a stem cell transplant? I knew she was under some stress.

On Saturday, February 20, my mother arrived in Orlando from Dallas. I was to check in to the hospital on February 23, and I had about five days of "freedom" from any needles or doctors. I made the two-and-a-half-hour drive to Orlando to pick her up. She was going to be there for the whole process. She hadn't even bought a return ticket yet. Her job was a unique one as a caregiver. She was the designated "kid entertainer." My mother is unique. She has never met a stranger. In fact, she became friends with a couple down the hall from us that had a dog, which my two youngest ones loved. My mother got to know them, found out their schedule for walking the dog, and made it a point to have Matthew and Amelia there to talk and pet the dog. It was little things like that that my mother was great at, keeping their minds on other things, walking a little bit of life with them. I don't think the kids understood the gravity of the transplant, but my mother did. My mother's assistance with our family helped my wife focus on being at the hospital.

While my wife was at the hospital several hours a day with me, my mother attended the kids, taking them to the clubhouse, to lunch, playing cards. It had become routine every night after supper to go to the clubhouse and have a "Thirty-one" tournament. That's a card game, by the way. Having my mother there to help Rhonda with the kids was nothing short of a miracle. No one under twelve was allowed in the hospital. My mother was a tremendous help, one that I will never be able to express in words.

I was released from the hospital on March 9, 2016. I was not able to go back home to Georgia at this time. We still needed to be near the hospital for the next month for blood work and doctor visits. My wife was planning a return back to Georgia for a week. My dad was flying in on March 12 for a week as the caregiver called up for relief. My dad arrived two days later at the Jacksonville airport for his relief work.

Now my dad arrived to give my wife some much-needed time to take care of other things. My dad sure did want to be there while I was in the hospital, but with the technology of phones, pictures, and Facetime, he was up to date the whole way. However, nothing replaces being there in person. For the next week, he would take me to the doctor, cook, entertain, and be a dad, just as if I was a little boy again.

I had an episode the first Sunday he was there. What I mean by that is, I was unable to keep supper down. It didn't happen often, but because of the chemotherapy, my stomach had some trouble digesting certain foods. He would make foods that were easy to digest, taking great care with what was being made for me to eat. I could tell he didn't like to see me not feeling well. As he would say many times, it sure beat the way I had been.

Even though I would not wish to do this again, we had some good times together. Sickness does that to people. We took some time to take long rides along the Florida coast, stopping along the way to observe the beaches, the sunsets, and much more. My mother and dad put forth a lot of effort, giving up some precious time of their life to help give care. It is important to have caregivers to help you through a serious medical treatment. I know many don't have what I had. I pray that the Lord will help them through the difficult process of treatment to see his good hand in their life.

Finally, there is my wife. I do not have words for her sacrifice, care, and kindness that she gave. There is way too much to write about here, and it would get boring to read. In a nutshell, she stood by me "in sickness and in health," a promise she'd made on April 11, 1992. It was now a reality. She managed to school our kids, cook, plan, prepare, play taxi, and too many other items to list. She also worked during this time. She is self-employed and works from home, but it is still work. It doesn't seem as if she ever missed a beat.

I have spent over half my life with this dear woman. She never complained, not one time. If I needed something, she got it. Proverbs 18:22 says, *"He who finds a wife finds a good thing, And obtains favor from the Lord."* I am thankful to this day that the favor of the Lord was upon me. Thank you, Rhonda, for being who you are.

As important as the treatment of your disease is, those around you who give up their time, plans, and freedom to be committed to caring for you during treatment are invaluable. Knowing that I had people there to help me was something I will never forget. Thank you all.

Post-Transplant Life

On May 19, 2016, I went back to work at United Parcel Service (UPS), where I am a service provider. In other words, I drive the brown truck. It is a physical job. Doing this job prior to my diagnosis with POEMS syndrome had become difficult. So this day means a lot to me. For a time, I thought I would not be able to do the job I loved to do. Being able to put on the brown uniform again was an accomplishment achieved only by the grace of God.

Post-transplant life is different. You think differently about everything. Where you eat, what you eat, who you are around, what you touch. Your own home is a bacteria trap as well. The toothpaste tube that you share with your spouse or kids? They may have rubbed their toothbrush on the tube, thus transferring any infecting germs to your toothbrush when you do the same. Those are things you always think about. You just don't want to get sick. At the very least, you do all you can *not* to get sick.

There were times where I might have been too cautious, but I don't think you can be too cautious in a post-transplant life. As time goes by, it gets better. Your immune system builds, and your white blood counts rise in order to respond to infection. Your body gets stronger, more like it used to be. The issue for most of us is time—we just don't like the waiting.

Some Cautious Thoughts

The doctors will give you guidelines to follow post transplant. The first 90 days is the benchmark. Regular blood tests are necessary, as often as three times a week. This is the time when you have to be the most careful. By being careful, I am talking about where you go, what you touch, and what you do. I speak from experience by saying that my body responded well and quickly, but it did not take long to realize I was not fully recovered. My strength didn't last long, even though I thought it would. I went back to work right at the 90-day post-transplant mark. I felt great. I went back on a Thursday, worked Friday and was glad the weekend was here. I was totally exhausted. I needed both of those days to recover.

Eating foods now is a concern. The guidelines and advice you will get in post-transplant instructions will advise you about which foods are good and which are not. In other words, don't eat sushi. Don't get shredded cheese out of the bag that six or seven other people have put their hands into. The same goes with chips. Get your own bag. Buffets are out of the question with food sitting out and hundreds of people breathing over it. Those glass shields? They don't work that well, in my opinion. One of my favorite places to eat is a sandwich shop. After careful study, with their foods and meats being slid all around and sitting out, I stayed away.

Large crowds such as those at church should be avoided for a while. The amount of people, contact, and folks wanting to shake your hand can create an easy path to infection. After a while, when you do go to church, carry a bottle of hand sanitizer with you, and use it...a lot. I have to trust that others will understand and not be offended if I apply the sanitizer after we shake hands. Movie theaters, malls, and public restrooms are places to be careful in, and ATM buttons and shopping carts are items to be careful with. Many, many people touch these, and whatever they have touched, you just touched.

Do not think you are being overly cautious. You're not. After all, it is your body, your health. Wipe items down and keep sanitizing hand wipes with you. When others drive your car, wipe down the keys, steering wheel, door handle, and gearshift.

If you plan to travel via airplane, this should be considered with great care. An airplane's circulating air system can carry things from the rear to the front and back again. I did fly eight weeks post transplant. It was risky. However, managing risk is all that you can do. I wore a mask the whole time in the airport and on the plane. The good thing about being a man who's nearly bald from chemo and wearing a mask at an airport is that you get special treatment. Those long security lines? Nope, you get ushered to the side and go through quickly. Remember to think about the "what-ifs" that may happen. It is far better to be safe than sorry.

Mind-Set As You Move Forward

I believe it is not out of the spiritual realm that attitude has some effect in recovery. I am not a "positive-thinker theology" man, but I do believe that an attitude of trusting in a faithful God is beneficial. I do struggle at times with the "what-ifs" of a disease. What if it shows signs of remission, which it could. What if I have to have another stem cell transplant? Yet I have decided that I'm going forward with the time God has granted me. Don't waste it, and don't allow Satan to steal your joy in God. All things are vanity here "under the sun," as Ecclesiastes tells us. But do not let that stop you from enjoying and pressing on under the sun.

Every day that you live post transplant is a goal accomplished. I did not have any serious infections. A slight sinus drainage about two months post transplant was all, and that was corrected by allergy medicine. Every day that you feel good is another accomplishment. I didn't always feel great, strong, and energetic every day, but as time progressed, I improved.

There were days I would see movements in my feet and experience feeling in my legs and a strength that I did not have previously. I would attempt to run, but that was still a problem. I would say, "I could not do this a year ago" and rejoice that I could now. These are some of the small things that you see. These are the things that measure your progress. The improvements you see help you march on to getting even better.

I don't want to be a wet blanket, but there are times when the fear of reoccurrence, or some other medical issues, arises. I have wrestled with this for some time. The fact is we are all dying, whether we're healthy or not. Having your hope planted in the foundation of God's truth helps you to press on for his glory each day. I think often of James 4:15, *"If the Lord wills, we will live and do this or that."* I have much to do now—work, play, minister, and get on the tractor. So I choose not to worry about what may or may not come. There is an indescribable amount of peace about that.

Helping Others

I was speaking to a nurse one day, and we were talking about a person's mind-set when it comes to dealing with health issues. I am convinced that God is both healer and sustainer of our lives. He uses man to discover healing medicines and treatments. However, behind all of man's knowledge is a sovereign God. I am also convinced that an attitude of hope makes a difference. I have seen some people give up, with no desire to get through the tough parts of a treatment, only to become weaker and have a great difficulty recovering.

Another way of encouraging and helping people deal with health issues is a forum I found very useful, **smartpatients.com**. This is a site where you can post questions and receive responses from many others who have been through or are going through similar situations. You can learn firsthand experience about others who have gone through similar situations. I found the forum very helpful as well when I had questions or struggles. There are many regulars on this site who provided coaching and encouragement, as those downtimes do hit when you're going through treatments. Or they can help you on that moment and day when the depression hits. For example, when my post recovery was not "panel perfect" (blood work perfect), then I hit a snag in my emotional health. It was here that others said their own blood work wasn't perfect, either, that it was now fluctuating or had fluctuated. Hearing from others who had the same "snags" in recovery helped me press on.

Preparing For Work

When you're preparing to go back to work, the criteria depend entirely upon what your job entails. My job was that of a delivery driver who was up and down many times a day. The average day was ten hours. Considering this, I felt good enough to work, but after two days, when I returned home, I was spent.

Getting back to work was, to me, the biggest milestone I could reach. It was huge for my emotional health. Given the fact that I was barely able to get up and down in my delivery truck just eight months prior, it was a miracle. My goal all along was to be back at work. God is good.

To be honest, my diagnosis came earlier than a lot of people with POEMS syndrome received theirs. So if your diagnosis has come later, then the improvements may take longer. But wait, trust, and let your body heal. Take those little steps. After all, it is only time.

Depending on your job, the amount of time that you will need to fully recover may vary. From my personal experience, physical activity is essential to a healthy recovery. I know that many won't feel like doing any physical work or exercise, but your body responds and you will be surprised how well you feel by doing it. You can push too far, but your body will know when it is time to quit.

Living In Your Post-Transplant World

You are a unique person, having had a bone marrow transplant. You are a child again, or your immune system is, anyway. The world you live in now is just as sick, viral, and germ ridden as it was before, yet you are most open to infection. Given this fact, you need to find a routine in your life to make it as normal as you can. As blood tests return and you see your labs normalizing and staying normal, you can do more than you could the first three to six months post transplant.

I have developed a routine in my life that has stayed with me post transplant. I am still cautious about where I eat and what I touch. These habits will likely be with you forever, and it is not all that bad a thing, either.

About seven months post transplant, I developed a scratchy throat, cough, and a fever. I called my doctors at the Mayo and was advised to watch the fever. I took some allergy medicine the doctor recommended, and after a day off work, I improved. This was huge. My immune system was now fighting off infection. Glory.

Going Forward

The Bible teaches us, *"Being confident of this one thing, that he who began a good work in you will complete it until the day of Jesus Christ"* (Philippians 1:6). I believe this verse. I know it is absolute truth. However, living it in real life is a challenge. I know that God began a work in me when he saved me. I know he will complete it. Living with a disease that could return is not easy. The worry implants in my mind, yet I know that I should not worry. I find that living with this possibility of relapse is most difficult.

The word of God gives me hope that is not found in earthly things. My hope is centered in what is to come. The Bible teaches us that God has prepared a place for us, and we shall be with him eternally. We are just sojourners and strangers in this world. It is not our home. It seems with this mind-set in focus, we are to go through life knowing who is controlling all things.

Every day that I am able to work, I think back to the days I could hardly work. The pain, the struggle, the fear and then to the hospital, where I was for nearly three weeks. It doesn't really matter how bad a day may be now, it was seemingly worse then. I'm better now. I'm working, functioning, and doing things I was pained to do before. As each day goes by, I do live with the reality, and even fear, that I may have to battle again. I have friends right now who are going through such battles. I am not sure that we can ever fully escape the reality of fear, but we have the word of God to help us. In Psalms 34:4, we read, "*I sought the Lord, and he answered me and delivered me from all my fears.*" This verse has been a help to me in the recovery. As I think about it, my seeking is to be to the Lord, always, and I should tell him my fear. Yes, I do fear that I may have signs of a relapse. But I will seek the Lord. I will ask him to help me with what I fear. And he will.

A final thought as I process what I have been through. Romans 8:28 says, "*And we know that for those who love God all things work together for good, for those who are called according to his purpose.*" This verse is one that I quoted for years to people who were enduring life's trials. It is much easier to quote than to live. It is a popular verse but one that establishes the sovereignty of God in all things. As I look back upon the season I went through suffering with POEMS, I see that ALL things do work together. I haven't fully seen the whole purpose yet, but I am different. I also missed the most important part of this verse. That is the "we know" part. We do know that God works things out for his good.

Knowing this makes me a more focused person, most of the time. I see that what God gives, he does so graciously. I try to walk the remaining days of my life focused on what matters, eternal things. Solomon in the book of Ecclesiastes assures us that all is vanity here under the sun. And it is. Knowing this gives me great joy. Now I can enjoy what God has granted me, knowing that all of our earthly possessions will be left behind.

My focus now is not on things that don't matter but those things that do.

I press forward today, not knowing what lies ahead but knowing who makes tomorrow, and who controls and works all things together. Dealing with a disease is difficult, but having a sovereign God who is your father is supreme. God bless your journey, and may he keep you and help you.

THE SPIRITUAL SIDE

James 4:15 says, "*If the Lord wills, we will live and do this or that.*" I suppose this sums up our outlook on life. Ecclesiastes 8:8 says, "*No man has power to retain the spirit, or power over the day of death.*" It's clear that our life is, by all accounts, in the hands of God. He determines who lives and who dies, at what time and by what method. This is not meant to be dismal, but we all will die. According to Hebrews 9:27, "*And just as it is appointed for man to die once, and after that comes judgment.*"

Upon diagnosis with POEMS, I had been a believer for about 20 years. I am still growing in the faith, learning, and God is molding me and shaping me. As with a clay pot, the potter molds and shapes me. I've had my moments of doubt. My faith was dealt a blow about the mortality of life landing in my lap. Most of us don't think about death until we reach a point somewhere late in life, at least not in great detail. For us to say that we have "weak faith" because we get in a crisis is foolish, but for us to put our faith in our circumstances is equally as foolish. Where's the balance?

It's All for a Purpose

I know this sounds clichéd, but Romans 8:28 says, *"And we know that for those who love God all things work together for good, for those who are called according to his purpose."* I remember I used to tell people this when they had a particular trial in their life. Now I had to believe it. Putting the Scriptures into practice is much harder than simply telling them to others. I now had to believe what I have always preached. I am here to tell you it was not easy. I asked myself, "What's the purpose in this?" I didn't see it at the time. We hardly ever see the purpose of a trial at the time of the trial.

In the book of Ruth, Naomi and her husband went to Moab during a drought. They left their homeland of Judah. When Naomi's husband died, along with her two sons, her heart was set on home. Ruth made the commitment to journey with her, but it was not easy. Neither Ruth nor Naomi likely realized why they were making the journey, nor why Ruth was in the field of Boaz, but she was. God used terrible circumstances to redeem Ruth, by placing her in the field of Boaz. What a marvelous story of love, hope, joy, and redemption. God still works today in circumstances we view as painful.

In February of 2015, we sold our house that we had built in 1999. I was in the middle stages of POEMS disease (although I didn't know it at the time) and was on the downhill slide. My father-in-law said we could live with him while we built a house. He graciously decided to deed us some land to do so. What should have taken 30 days instead took 94 days, and at the time, I was anxious, knowing we needed to get started. We were looking at modular homes then decided we wanted a stick-built house. The plans were drawn up, but they took longer, and the land deed was still not done.

Now I began to get frustrated. Why was this taking so long? Why was the paperwork still sitting on the judge's desk? I also gave the plans to a friend at church who is a builder. He was taking a while to get his prices for us as well. In late July 2015, we had a trip planned to Colorado. While we were there with my parents from Texas, the conversation turned to my health. My parents were greatly concerned. Sitting on the couch in the room that week, I made the call to Johns Hopkins for an appointment, and the date was set for one month later.

What is important for us to grasp in our lives is that God is working things out, even when we don't see the plan. That's essentially how he works in our lives many times—behind the scenes. John Piper said, "God is always doing 10,000 things in your life, and you may be aware of three of them." God is at work even when we feel as if he is not. Looking back on events often helps us see God's hand in those events. The delays do not seem like delays but, instead, divine interventions. Seeing it then was tough, but seeing it now, we glorify God.

Seeing The Purpose

This is where things get tough, trusting that God has a plan that he has not revealed to you yet. Leaving the grounds of comfort for the grounds of promise. Being positive, uplifting, and encouraging are qualities that do play a part in the healing and recovery process. But they are not the foundation for the battle. It is extraordinarily difficult to see a purpose in sickness without the knowledge of God's will. Seeing God's will as a Christian is still difficult, though. Suffering for Christ is hard, although the Bible says we may endure such affliction.

Suffering in the Bible often referred to persecution for being a believer. In America today, we don't really understand the depths of this type of persecution. The suffering I endured was not by men from a communist or dictatorial government. It was from an affliction of sickness. Yet does this type of suffering have a greater good? Does physical persecution from government extremists have a good? Yes, they all do. Seeing it becomes the great challenge before us.

Sickness was not uncommon in the ancient days. Today we have many great medical advancements to help with even the very common illnesses that killed people in years past. In the New Testament, we see that many were sick and had fevers. Sickness was not uncommon. And God used many of these instances of healing to show who he truly is, to prove and give an example of God coming in the flesh. The Bible is full of such miracles, too many to begin listing here.

Back to Romans 8:28 and me trying to define what *"all*

things work together for the good" means. I suppose that there are sufferings that we may never see the good in here on earth. This is why we don't have our hearts set on earth. Colossians 3:2 says, *"Set your minds on things that are above, not on things that are on earth."* Setting your mind is like an airplane setting its heading. Once set, the airplane will fly in that direction. It has a course set. For the believer, the course is set to heaven. As Paul says in Philippians 3:14, *"I press on toward the goal for the prize of the upward call of God in Christ Jesus."* By pressing on, he has set the course. Understanding Romans 8:28 helps us grasp our spiritual heading. If we're pressing toward heaven, then no matter what happens, it is for our good. If we're healed, we win, and if we're not, we win. Either way, it is for our good. I believe this is how we get understanding in the purpose of sickness and suffering. Where's our heading?

Not A Defined Reason But Trust

God does not have to give us a reason for our suffering. God does not have to explain anything to us. We have to elevate our way of thinking in forms of trust. We must trust God in all that we encounter, whether that is a physical suffering in a hostile nation or a suffering in our lives in a free nation. God is sovereign. Proverbs 3:5,6 says, *"Trust in the Lord with all your heart, and do not lean on your own understanding. In all your ways acknowledge him, and he will make straight your paths."* I never thought much about the *"in all your ways,"* but that means the same as Romans 8:28's *"all things,"* and for me, this is where the foundation of trust begins. In all that we endure, we trust God because he is good, faithful, sovereign, and eternal.

Trusting God is like trusting your father or mother as a young child. You know they will take care of you. You have confidence that you can jump off the kitchen counter and your father will catch you. The fact is, you never really doubt that he will. With God as our father, we should jump and know he will catch us.

Psalms mentions trust 53 times. Evidently the writers of the Psalms knew something about trusting in God, given the fact that they were often pursued by enemies. Psalms 20:7 defines where our trust should be: "*Some trust in chariots and some in horses, but we trust in the name of the Lord our God.*" Material things are not eternal. They do not grant peace or respond to our request, but God does. Trusting God in times of difficulty is not easy. Why? Because we want it our way. I have learned that he knows best. He sees more than I see and is orchestrating events to accomplish his will.

Trusting God when you can't see the outcome is not easy. No spiritual giant can ever tell me different. I know I should trust God in every situation, and I think I do, but there are times when it takes a while to trust. I often try to sort and work things out for myself. God has a plan. I know that sounds clichéd, but it's true. He does. We sow grass but don't see immediate results. We want immediate results, but it takes time.

Dealing With The Outcome

We all want to be healed, but we are all dying. Every healthy person, even one with no issues at all, is dying. Romans 5:12 says, *"Therefore, just as sin came into the world through one man, and death through sin, and so death spread to all men because all sinned."* All men are sinners, dying without the redemption of Christ. According to Romans 5:15, *"For if many died through one man's trespass, much more have the grace of God and the free gift by the grace of that one man Jesus Christ abounded for many."* Given these Scriptures, we know that men are dying, but the saving grace is Christ and our belief in him.

Understanding the outcome for the Christian is vital to our spiritual walk. For example, one who is not physically healed of cancer or disease here on earth is eternally healed because they are with the Lord. One who is physically healed of disease or cancer here on earth is healed to tell the story of God's grace. As of summer 2017, my disease is in remission. Every 90 days I go for blood work and tests. I get a little nervous awaiting those tests. Who wouldn't? For some reason, the Lord has spared my earthly life. He has put me in a job where I see a lot of people. Some of those people are dealing with sickness and disease. There I am given opportunity to share my story. Many are encouraged as they see me working, and they know that God will work all things to the good.

For now, friends, I will enjoy the healing God has given me. I will press on in my daily walk, seeking opportunity to share the story God has given me. This story is one God has worked out for the good. I didn't see the good two years earlier in all the delays, but he did. Trusting God's hand in directing our lives through suffering, sickness, and persecution is not something you can do if you're not one of his. We endure because we are his.

A JOURNEY IN PICTURES

A picture is worth a thousand words. Actions speak louder than words. Defining moments in our life are often captured in photos. Looking at old photos brings back great memories of childhood holidays or events in your life. It takes you back to a time that you often remember so vividly. I have many old pictures stuffed away that I bring out from time to time. And it brings me back to that moment in my life when things were different. Amazing things photos are. Oh how precious memories are. We see photos where we had no idea what the next months, weeks, or years would bring.

Photos tell great stories. A photo captures moments in time. Seeing an old photo helps you to remember where you were at. For me, seeing these pictures reminds me of how God has worked. It is physical proof that he is in control of life and death.

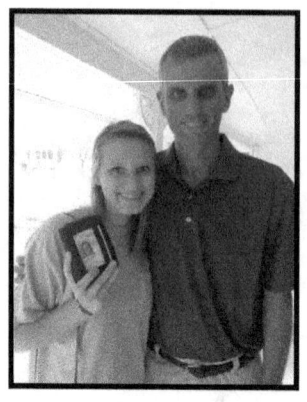

The Picture That Made Me Realize I Was Sick, Really Sick

This was the day my second daughter received her driver's license. My wife took the picture, we looked at it, and the look on her face was astounding. She knew I was sick. I saw at that moment how bad I looked. I would look in the mirror and see my arms looking small. I have never been a small guy. In fact, my arms were almost as small as my wife's. She's 110 pounds and has a small frame. I was secretly worried. It wasn't getting any better.

From January 2015 through the late summer of 2015, people began to notice. I was having trouble with stairs. I would ask my children to help me carry a plate of food because I had to use both hands to climb two stairs. I had an appointment at

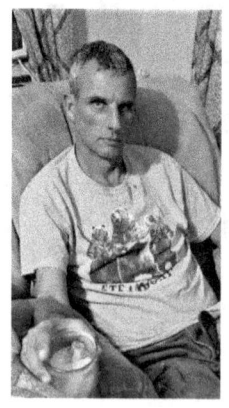

Johns Hopkins in late August, and this picture was taken in mid-August. The timing was right. Much longer and I would likely have been in seriously worse shape.

October 2015 - Treatment Beginning

Weighing in at 178 pounds and the day I started the oral chemo pill. I remember this day all too well. That ole chair, which has since been decommissioned. It was my comfort spot. That chair had been with us for many years. Once a prime seat in the living room of our old house, it made its way to the man cave in our basement. The treatment plan was in order. I remember having hope of its success at this time. I'm thankful to the Lord it was. I was glad to be taking this treatment. I was at peace. I had comfort. The relief of knowing and attacking the disease was a huge weight off my shoulders. Now to get better.

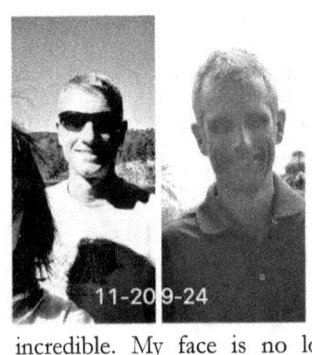

The Transformation

After I started oral chemo, my wife and I had a weekend in the North Georgia Mountains. We snapped this picture less than two months after initial treatment. The transformation is incredible. My face is no longer sunk in, my skin color is different, and I have some weight gain. I cannot describe in words how I felt at this time, looking in the mirror and seeing the Lord work a miracle. I felt better. I thought better. I didn't hurt as much. I was walking better.

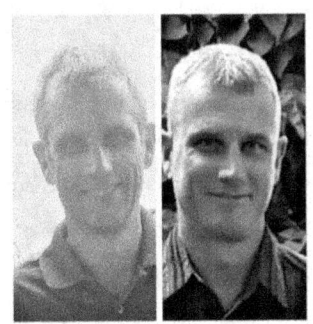

This picture shows a two and a half month difference.

On the left was the first trip to the Mayo Clinic. The one on the right was my two month follow up after starting chemo.

The Florida hat was not my personal choice. I'm a Texas Longhorns fan. But there are no Texas hats in Jacksonville. Plus the gator hat is bright and happy. This was the day of dismissal, a

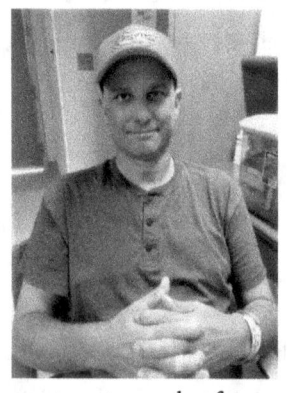

day I had hoped for. Finally it was here. I felt at this moment as if a huge hill had been climbed. I knew that there might be some weak days ahead. But I was out of the hospital.

Yahtzee became the game for us while staying post transplant in Jacksonville. We stayed at the apartment complex for an additional month after being released from the hospital. Pictured with me is my son, the last of four, who was seven years old at the time. My parents, my wife, and

my kids all played Yahtzee at the poolside. It was a relaxing time for us as we patiently endured the recovery.

I was still making twice weekly trips to the Mayo for blood work to see the progress of cells rebuilding. I don't believe it rained a single time, at least not for more than a

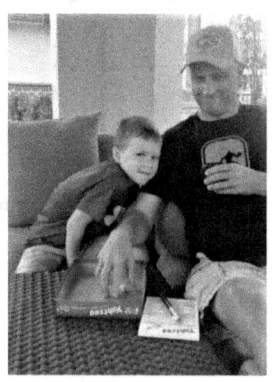

few minutes, while we were there. This gave us ample time to go to the beach, to ride the back roads as we passed the time. It was a time I won't soon forget.

As you can see, I ditched the Florida Gators hat. My dad, who flew in for relief work again, brought some real Texas hats.

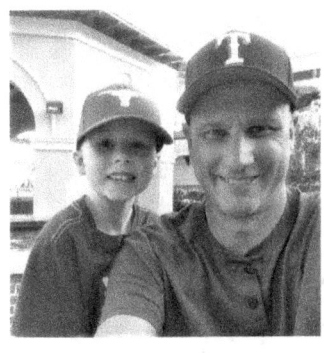

He knew I would be lacking proper foliage on the head. I still have these hats. And every time I put them on it reminds me of these days. I love photos. They bring you to a place of remembrance. I don't want to ever forget these days, seeing where the Lord has brought me from and hoping I don't ever go back. However, God remains in control. He always has been and always will be.

POSTSCIPT

I've learned some valuable lessons since enduring this trial that began in the middle of 2013. As of this writing, it is fall of 2017. Four years later and what have I learned? Not so much what have I learned but what can I share looking back over the process that will help encourage you who may be facing a diagnosis and trial?

Living with the fear of reoccurrence is a battle I face quite a bit. So I have decided that I cannot worry about what may happen. A tree may fall on me while walking in the woods. I don't want that to keep me from hiking, therefore, I won't worry about that. I take the same approach to any disease that may arise—again, *may* arise. Spending time worrying about all the possibilities will not help. Enjoy the day.

Help and encourage others when you have the opportunity. I make at least four trips a year to the Mayo Clinic. I am in the follow-up stages. I see people there who seem to be in the diagnosis stages. I have been able, while in the waiting area or cafeteria, to strike up conversations. I tell them of the miracle that God has given me. I share what I faced. I try to encourage them that they are in the best place this side of heaven. That as I have tried to learn, that *"All things work together"* from Romans 8:28 is real. It is a constant work in my life, but I see it becoming more of a reality.

Whatever stage you are in of your diagnosis, treatment, or recovery, look ahead and not behind. I'm confident because of Philippians 1:6, *"And I am sure of this, that he who began a good work in you will bring it to completion at the day of Jesus Christ."* Furthermore, Philippians 3:14 says, *"I press on toward the goal for the prize of the upward call of God in Christ Jesus."* Considering that our life is not that lengthy at all, I cherish the great hope God has granted me of eternal life. Sick or healthy, we won't live forever here.

Take a look around and see the beauty of God. Look and see the working of God in all things. See the waiting room where God uses men to heal through advances in medicine. And glorify God for all that. Bless his name for being intimately involved in the daily lives we live. I try to keep Psalms 34:1 in my heart at all times: *"I will bless the Lord at all times; his praise shall continually be in my mouth."*

May the Lord bless your health and healing in the journey you're on.

ABOUT THE AUTHOR

Brad L Horton is a bi-vocational pastor of Mt. Carmel Baptist Church in Temple, Georgia. He is married to Rhonda, they have four kids ranging from 22 to 9. Brad is employed with UPS as a driver, likes piddling around their farm, reading, writing and is an avid aviation hobbyist. Most of all, his passion is the exposition of God's word that he does each week.